NUTRITIONAL MYTHS – EXPOSED#

-EAT THIS NOT THAT-

RAW TRUTH ABOUT ALL TRADITIONAL NUTRITIONAL MYTHS

PREFACE

WE ALL WANT TO BE HEALTHY TODAY.EVERY BODY FOLLOWING SOME MYTHS TO KEEP THEM HEALTHY AND STRONG.FEW PEOPLE FOLLOW SOME MYTHS BLINDLY TO REDUCE WEIGHT.BUT THEY DON'T EVER ASK A DOCTOR OR NUTRINITIST WHETHER ITS CORRECT OR NOT.THEY JUST FOLLOWING AS THEY ARE BEING TOLD BY SOME CLOSE FRIEND OR RELATIVES.IN THIS BOOK IM GOING TO CLER ALL THE DOUBTS ABOUT THE NUTRITIONAL MYTHS.ARE THEY TRUE OR NOT.MAY BE YOU ARE FOLLOWING RIGHT ONE MAY BE TOTALLY WRONG...............

DEDICATION

THIS BOOK IS ENTIRELY DEDICATED TO THE DEVINE POWER "LORD KRISHNA".

-"JAY SHRI KRISHNA"-

<u>INTRODUCTION</u>

Are you overwhelmed by daily decisions about what to eat, how much to eat, when to eat, and how much physical activity you need to be healthy? If so, don't be discouraged because you're not alone. With so many choices and decisions, it can be hard to know what to do and which information you can trust.

This information in this book may help you make changes in your daily eating and physical activity habits so that you improve your well-being and reach or maintain a healthy weight.

WHAT IS MYTH?

According to Wikipedia Myth is a folklore genre consisting of narratives or stories that play a fundamental role in a society, such as foundational tales or origin myths.

Another definition of Myth is a widely held but false belief or idea.

The myths those are related to nutritional facts are Nutritional Myths.

There are so many nutritional myths are there. Some of them are true and some are totally false. In this book I will discuss about some very common myths regarding health and nutrition.

After reading and understanding, the choices will be yours.

MYTH NUMBER 1#

Eating after 8 p.m causes weight gain and obesity.

The natural principle of our body metabolism is Calories in= Calories out and the quantity and type of food matters to our body weight.

Time is not the thing which matters, it's all about quality and quantity of eating which intern controls your body weight.

So try to eat healthy irrespective of time and avoid mindless eating to avoid obesity.

MYTH NUMBER 2#

EGG YOLK IS BAD FOR YOU AND IT CAUSES CHOLESTEROL

You used to hear that eating whole egg causes heart disease by elevating body's cholesterol level.egg yolk is the main kalprit,so avoid it and take only egg white.

I would like to say that this myth is a totally wrong one. The cholesterol in egg increases HDL cholesterol level in blood which in term is good cholesterol. This HDL helps in peripheral fat mobilization and it's a key ingredient in brain. Apart from cholesterol an boiled egg also contains sodium,potassium,protein(biotin),so me vitamins like A,D,C,B-6. Iron and cobalamine also present in egg.

American heart association is telling that whole egg have no relations with congestive or ischemic heart disease or even uncontrolled hypertension.

If you take a whole boiled egg regularly in the breakfast then your hunger urges will be reduced as it contains healthy fats and thus it helps in calorie cutting and weight loss.

Eat egg regularly…….

MYTH NUMBER 3#

ONE SHOULD EAT 5-7 SMALLER MEALS A DAY TO KEEP THE METABOLISM TICKING AND THUS REDUCE OR CONTROLE WEIGHT

In this case you have to understand the TDEE which is TOTAL DAILY ENERGY EXPENDITURE. It is the sum of B.M.R(basal metabolic rate)+Activity level+Thermic effect of food.

BMR-it is the energy expenditure at resting state of body

ACTIVITY LEVEL-is the sum of works you do in a day.

THERMIC EFFECT OF FOOD-it is the energy required to digest the food you take, which is about 10% of the total calories you take by food in a day. This is constant.

For example, if you take 2000 calories in a day then your TDEE will be 200 calories. So you take 2 meals or 8 meals that will not going to change your daily TDEE.

So this small frequent meal system won't help you in metabolism to lose your weight.

It is seen in many researches that the people who are taking 2 major meals compared with the peoples who are taking 7-8 small meals have no differentiation in weight loss protocol.

<u>MYTH NUMBER 4#</u>

<u>SALT SHOULD BE RESTRICTED IN ORDER TO AVOID HEART DISEASE OR HYPERTENSION.</u>

Common salt or sodium hydrochloride retain water inside the body by reabsorbing at kidney level so it increases your blood pressure by 1-5mmHg only on an average. By this a normal individual cannot get a hypertensive disorder or heart problems.

But if you have any medical conditions like salt sensitive hypertension or chronic dyslipidaemia(increased bad cholesterol level in blood) or chronic kidney disease then your arteries are at risk and you should restrict salt intake from your diet according to your doctor's advice.

But a normal healthy individual should not cut the normal salt intake via food as it may bring some medical emergencies like acute hyponatraemia(sudden fall of blood sodium).

The American Heart Association recommends no more than 2300 mg a day is the standard requirement of salt for adults. For children it is not more than 1500mg/day.

MYTH NUMBER 5#

WHOLE WHEAT IS A HEALTHY FOOD AND IT IS AN ESSENTIAL PART OF A 'BALANCED DIET'

Wheat has been a part of the diet for a very long period of time. But it is changed due to genetic tampering in the 1960's.From that time the new wheat becomes less nutritious than the old one.

Few studies have shown that compared to the older wheat, the modern wheat may increase the level of bad cholesterol by carbohydrate overdose and it also contains some inflammatory markers which produces symptoms like joint pain,aches,irritable bowel syndrome. This eventually changes the quality of individuals' lifestyle in long run.

The market is saturated now with refined white and flour. These things have no effect in weight loss but definitely on weight gain.

MYTH NUMBER 6#

COFFEE IS TOXIC/UNHEALTHY AND SHOULD BE AVOIDED

A major portion of society thinks that coffee is unhealthy and should not be taken throughout the year.

But a very small group only knows that coffee is one of the biggest sources of antioxidants out ranking the fruits and vegetables.

Regular black coffee drinkers have much lower risk of depression,anxiety,alzhimers,perkins onism and many other psychosomatic illness.

So don't forget to take a coffee break unless you have a coffee triggering migraine attack history.

MYTH NUMBER 7#

EATING FAT MAKES YOU FATTY.AVOID ALL FATS

All fats are not bad. There are two types of fat, one is saturated and another is unsaturated fat.

The saturated type fats are the bad ones and this is present in high quantity in fatty lamb/beef/pork, butter/cheese etc.

But the mono and polyunsaturated fats are good for your health which presents in olive oil, canola oil, peanut oil, sesame oil, corn oil etc.

This unsaturated variety helps your brain and other organs to function normally.

So avoid bad fat sources, not the good ones.

MYTH NUMBER 8#

A HIGH PROTEIN DIET CAUSES STRESS OVER KIDNEY AND MAY LEAD TO KIDNEY DISEASE

High protein diet is only restricted in established chronic kidney disease or renal failure or hyperuricemic patients, because high protein produces an abnormal solute load over kidney only in above mentioned medical conditions.

But as a normal individual you can take as much protein as an athelet.high protein lowers the blood pressure and fight against type 2 diabetes mellitus. Protein reduces appetite which intern helps in weight loss.

Our muscular system is totally made up of proteins. High protein intake maintain adequate muscle health.

<u>MYTH NUMBER 9#</u>

<u>LOW FAT FOODS ARE HEALTHY BECAUSE THEY ARE LOWER IN CALORIES AND NO SATURATED FATS</u>

When the low-fat guideline first came out, the food manufacturers responded with all sorts of low-fat 'healthy foods'. But the problem is-these foods tests horrible when the fat is removed from them. So the food manufacturers added a whole bunch of sugar instead.

This extra sugar is very much harmful while the fat naturally present in the food is not.

So always remember that processed low fat foods tend to be very high in sugar compared to the natural fatty foods.

<u>MYTH NUMBER 10#</u>

REFINED OILS ARE PURE AND CHOLESTEROL FREE COMPARED TO THE MUSTARD OIL BECAUSE THEY ARE GOOD FOR HEART AND HEALTH

This is a complete misconcepeption.any natural oil like pure /virgin mustard oil, corn oil,oliv oil,soyabin oil etc are rich in Omega 6 polyunsaturated fatty acid which lower the level of cholesterol level in blood. But the refined oils are completely chemical in nature. Because refined oils undergoes so many chemical process like heating at very high temperature, chemical bleaching so as to make it transparent and odor free.tn this very process all the vital ingredients'/nutrients are lost. So we are taking chemical in the form of refined oils. There is no oil property present in this type oils and in term they causes many disease like obesity,osteoporosis,high blood sugar, and even cancer.

<u>MYTH NUMBER 11#</u>

PROTEIN TAKES CALCIUM AWAY FROM YOUR BONE AND PROMOT OSTEOPOROSIS

This is a common thought that eating high protein raises the acidity of the blood and take out calcium from the bone which may cause osteoporosis. Although it is true that a high protein intake increases calcium excretion in the short term but this effect does not persist in the long term.

The truth is that a high protein intake is linked to a massively reduced risk of osteoporosis and old age stress fractures.

Numerous studies are available that eating high protein is linked to a reduced risk of osteoporosis and fracture.

Don't cut protein unless you have some medical conditions like hyperuricaemia,CKD,kidney failure etc.

<u>MYTH NUMBER 12#</u>

LOSING WEIGHT IS ALL ABOUT WILL POWER AND EATING LESS WITH LOTS OF EXERCISE

All folks think that weight loss is all about calories in v/s calories out.

But unfortunately this is not the fact.

Our body is very complex structure which is controlled by numerous factors like brain energy, mental health, hormonal secretions and regulations, biological clock. All this factors controls body weight also.

If you only focus on calories and you are suffering from an undiagnosed psycho-somatic illness like panaxic depressive disorders, which in term producing a negative impact on your mind,brain,body,hormones then you just can't lose weight rather you will gain weight.

Please do not cut calories without proper understanding or by seeing some videos in YouTube or google.Take expert's consultation.

This is also applicable for your exercise prescription.

You are 90 kegs and your height is 5.3 ft and you just starts morning moderate running by seeing a Google reference, then you are damaging your knee cartilages. Soon you will get knee and heel pain.

So before doing exercise also you have to consults an expert.

MYTH NUMBER 13#

RED MEAT IS THE SOURCE OF HEART DISEASE AND TYPE 2 DIABETES

There two types of meat available in the market.

Fresh and unprocessed

Processed meat

The second one is the poison.

As it contains many preservative chemicals. But the fresh cooked meats are beneficial for health.

Please do not overcook as it causes protein denaturation and may be harmful.

So in one word processed overcooked deep fried meats are not healthy.

MYTH NUMBER 14#

CEREBRAL STROK OR CVA IS THE RESUALT OF ABNORMAL ACIDITY AND GAS FORMATION

This is typically an Indian myth and is totally a misconceptation.

Whenever you eat a biogas called methane is formed inside the intestine and stomach which leaves body per rectal way.

If you have gastritis or acidity then you may experience abdominal discomfort but it does not have any relations with CVA.

CVA is the result of chronic uncontrolled hypertensive crisis.

Gastritis, excessive abdominal gas formation or acidity has no role in cerebral or cardiogenic attack.

MYTH NUMBER 15#

AFTER 45 YRS OF AGE YOU NEED DAILY CALCIUM SUPPLIMENTS

After 45 calcium is needed.

But first assess the requirement of your body calcium and the take supplements' unless your requirement is served. Then just stop taking pills of calcium carbonate because it may not be absorbed by your bones and get deposited in the organ like kidney or gallbladder.

Then you will get a gallstone for free with the calcium pills.

Another thing,focous on taking cholecalciferol or vit D3 along with calcium pills for proper absorption .

MYTH NUMBER 16#

BREAD IS BAD AND IF YOU EAT THEN EAT ONLY WHOLE WHEAT BREAD OR BROWN BREAD

The anti bread fellows(those who don't eat bread and don't allow anyone to eat bread!)generally makes two arguments against bread consumption-

1.bread will make you fat

2.bread contains lots of gluten, which is poison for human

Only bread will never make you fat.we people eat bread always withhigh calorie foods like butter, jam,etc.

This leads to a calorie surplus and thus the result is weight gain.

So we should bread only with fruits and veggis.then it will not be a problem.

The gluten is problem only in Celiac Disease as it triggers an immune response in them which damages the lining of small intestine. So avoid bread only you are gluten sensitive or suffering from Celiac Disease.

END